BATTEN DISEASE DIET

Complete Diet Guide To Manage,
Understanding, Planning, And
Implementing Nutritional Strategies For
Better Health And Well-Being

Dr. Holmgren Alfred

A beacon of knowledge, "Batten Disease Diet: With Expert Guidance" is a thorough and invaluable resource for people and families navigating the complexities of Batten Disease.

It provides expert insights and useful advice catered to the specific dietary needs of those affected by this difficult condition.

Fundamentally, the book explores the causes, symptoms, and progression of Batten disease; however, it goes beyond this and acknowledges the critical role that nutrition plays in managing the disease, underscoring the significant influence that nutrition can have on general health and wellbeing.

Readers are guided step-by-step into the field of nutritional science and emerge with a deep comprehension of the essential nutrients needed to manage Batten's Disease. Every component—from vitamins to minerals and antioxidants—is carefully analyzed, enabling readers to make well-informed dietary decisions.

The Battens Disease diet planning and execution chapters combine practicality and precision, giving readers the tools to assess their own nutritional needs, create balanced meal plans, and navigate the finer points of meal preparation and portion control.

Beyond theory, the book provides a wealth of nutrient-rich food options that are specifically tailored to support optimal health in Battens Disease patients.

But it's not just about what to eat; it's also about what not to eat. Readers are guided through the maze of dietary pitfalls, equipped with knowledge to manage potential allergies and sensitivities and avoid foods and substances that may aggravate symptoms.

The book emphasizes the significance of staying hydrated by providing specific insights on how much fluids to drink and which beverages to choose.

It also discusses the various obstacles that both patients and caregivers must overcome, including how to manage gastrointestinal symptoms, swallowing issues, and changing dietary requirements as the disease progresses.

Supplements and drugs are discussed carefully and clearly, providing information on their functions, side effects, and standard advice.

In the meantime, helpful hints for caregivers are invaluable, providing assistance with meal preparation and planning as well as handling dietary restrictions and difficulties.

Beyond the boundaries of diet alone, the book embraces a holistic approach, exploring the interplay between lifestyle factors, physical activity, stress management, and complementary therapies.

As the journey continues, the importance of monitoring and adjusting the diet becomes apparent, ensuring that nutritional needs are met and deficiencies are addressed promptly.

"Batten Disease Diet: With Expert Guidance" is more than just a book; it's a reliable companion that helps people and caregivers navigate the complex web of Batten disease with kindness, lucidity, and resolute knowledge.

This book, "Batten Disease Diet: With Expert Guidance," contains information that should only be used for informational purposes. It is not meant to replace professional medical advice, diagnosis, or treatment. If you have any questions about a medical condition, you should always consult a physician or other qualified health provider.

While [Your Name], the book's author, has taken reasonable steps to ensure that the information is correct and current as of the publishing date, no express or implied representations or warranties are made regarding the availability, completeness, accuracy, reliability, suitability, or accuracy of the information contained in these pages.

You therefore use this material at your own risk and should not rely on it in any way. The author disclaims all liability for any loss, damage, or injury resulting from or related to the use of this book.

The author does not endorse any specific people, products, websites, organizations, or other names referenced or mentioned in this book; furthermore, any mention of names, products, websites, organizations, or other names within this book is purely informative and does not imply endorsement.

Before implementing any dietary or lifestyle modifications based on the information in this book, it is crucial to speak with a licensed healthcare provider, particularly if you have any underlying medical conditions or concerns.

CHAPTER 1
INTRODUCTION TO BATTEN DISEASE

Neuronal ceroid lipofuscinosis (NCL), another name for Batten disease, is a rare, inherited neurodegenerative disorder that mainly affects children. It is characterized by the build-up of lip pigments in the body's tissues, especially in the brain and nervous system. This leads to progressive neurological impairment, which includes cognitive decline, seizures, loss of motor skills, and ultimately early death. The disorder is brought on by genetic mutations that interfere with the normal function of lysosomes—cellular organelles that break down and recycle various molecules—which causes a build-up of toxic substances within cells, which in turn causes extensive damage and degeneration of neurons.

Knowing the Causes, Symptoms, and Progression of Batten disease

The majority of Batten disease cases are caused by mutations in the genes that encode proteins involved in lysosomal trafficking and degradation processes (CLN3, CLN5, CLN6, CLN7, and CLN8). These genetic defects impair the ability of lysosomes to break down cellular waste products, which leads to the accumulation of lip pigments within cells. Over time, this accumulation damages neurons and other cells throughout the body, resulting in the typical symptoms of Batten disease.

As the disease progresses, affected individuals may experience cognitive decline, loss of motor function, and behavioral changes. Ultimately, Batten disease leads to severe disability and premature death, usually by late adolescence or early adulthood.

The age of onset and severity can vary depending on the specific genetic mutation. Early signs may include developmental delays, vision loss, and seizures, which get worse over time.

There is currently no known cure for Batten disease, and available treatments are primarily aimed at managing symptoms and improving quality of life. The disease progresses relentlessly and irreversibly, with affected individuals experiencing a steady decline in neurological function over time as neurons continue to degenerate and die. Eventually, the symptoms become more severe and lead to profound physical and cognitive impairment.

Diet is Crucial for Managing Battens Disease:

While there is no known cure for Batten disease, managing symptoms and supporting overall health and well-being in affected individuals are greatly aided by proper nutrition; seizures, malnutrition, and gastrointestinal issues can all be mitigated by eating a well-balanced diet; certain dietary interventions may also help slow the disease's progression and improve quality of life for patients and their families.

Maintaining an adequate calorie intake to support growth and development is one of the most important nutritional considerations for people with Batten disease. Children who suffer from swallowing difficulties, gastrointestinal problems, or loss of appetite may find it difficult to eat, which puts them at risk for malnutrition and failure to thrive, both of which can accelerate the disease's progression.

Caregivers must collaborate closely with healthcare professionals, such as dietitians and feeding therapists, to make sure that affected individuals receive the nutrients and calories they need to support their particular needs.

Dietary composition is important for managing Batten disease in addition to calorie intake; some research indicates that certain nutrients, like antioxidants and omega-3 fatty acids, may have neuroprotective effects and help mitigate oxidative stress and inflammation in the brain; foods rich in antioxidants, like fruits, vegetables, and whole grains, may help reduce the accumulation of toxic substances and slow the progression of neurodegeneration in Batten disease; the cognitive function and brain health of these individuals has been demonstrated.

Additionally, dietary adjustments might be required to address particular symptoms and complications associated with Batten disease. For instance, people who have the disease frequently experience seizures, which could be made worse by blood sugar fluctuations. In these situations, a diet low in refined sugars and carbohydrates, like the ketogenic diet, could help stabilize blood sugar levels and lessen the frequency and severity of seizures. Similarly, dietary fiber and hydration are crucial for managing gastrointestinal symptoms, which are common in people with Batten disease and include reflux and constipation.

Despite the fact that there is presently no known cure for Batten disease, good nutrition is crucial for managing symptoms and promoting overall health and well-being in those who are afflicted. A balanced diet that offers enough calories, nutrients, and fluids can help reduce complications related to the disease and improve the quality of life for patients and their families. Caregivers must collaborate closely with healthcare providers to create customized meal plans that take into account the special requirements and difficulties of Batten disease. By using a comprehensive strategy that combines medical management, nutritional support, and supportive care, it is possible to maximize results and improve the quality of life for those who have the disease.

CHAPTER 2
ESSENTIALS OF A BATTENS DISEASE DIET

A bowel disease Diet is a customized approach to nutrition that aims to support overall health and potentially slow the progression of the disease. It recognizes the complex interplay between nutrition and neurological health and emphasizes the importance of specific nutrients and dietary guidelines in optimizing the well-being of individuals affected by Batten disease. Batten disease is an uncommon and fatal inherited disorder of the nervous system that presents a unique set of challenges that require careful management, including dietary considerations.

Summary Of Nutritional Objectives

The nutritional objectives of a diet for Batten's disease center on meet the various needs of the people who have the disease. These needs include:

(1) sustaining sufficient nutrition is critical to support general health and well-being because Battens disease can impair nutrient absorption and metabolism;

(2) optimizing neurological function by providing nutrients that support brain health and mitigate the degenerative effects of the disease;

(3) managing symptoms like seizures and muscle weakness through dietary interventions is a crucial component of the nutritional goals;

(4) ultimately improving quality of life and possibly lengthening survival by catering to the unique nutritional requirements of those with the disease.

Important Nutrients to Consider: Antioxidants, Minerals, and Vitamins

In the context of Batten disease, these nutrients take on extra importance because the disease affects metabolic processes and cellular integrity.

For example, vitamin E, a strong antioxidant, has been demonstrated to guard against oxidative stress-induced neuronal damage, which is especially pertinent in neurodegenerative disorders like Batten disease.

Similarly, minerals like calcium and magnesium are necessary for nerve conduction and muscle function, both of which may be impaired in Battens disease patients.

Therefore, focusing on a nutrient-rich diet that provides ample amounts of vitamins, minerals, and antioxidants is important.

Developing specific dietary guidelines for Batten disease management involves a comprehensive approach that takes into account individual needs, symptoms, and disease progression.

Firstly, maintaining a well-balanced diet that includes a variety of nutrient-dense foods is essential to meet overall nutritional requirements.

Emphasizing whole foods such as fruits, vegetables, lean proteins, and healthy fats can help provide essential nutrients while minimizing the intake of processed foods and added sugars, which offer little nutritional value and may exacerbate symptoms.

Additionally, considering the specific symptoms and complications associated with Batten's disease, dietary modifications may be necessary.

For example, individuals experiencing seizures may benefit from a ketogenic diet, which has been shown to reduce seizure frequency in certain neurological conditions. Furthermore, ensuring adequate hydration and managing swallowing difficulties, common issues in Batten disease, are integral components of dietary management.

Collaborating with healthcare professionals, including registered dietitians and neurologists, is essential in developing and implementing personalized dietary guidelines tailored to the unique needs of individuals with Batten disease.

a bowel disease Diet is a comprehensive nutritional strategy that supports neurological function, manages symptoms, and supports overall health. Individuals with Batten disease may benefit from improved long-term outcomes and quality of life if they follow dietary guidelines, incorporate personalized interventions, and concentrate on essential nutrients.

CHAPTER 3

CREATING A DIET PLAN FOR BATTEN DISEASE

People who have Battens Disease, also called neuronal ceroid lipofuscinosis (NCL), are primarily affected by this rare and inherited neurodegenerative disorder that progresses gradually, causing a range of symptoms such as vision loss, cognitive decline, and mobility issues. Since there is currently no cure for Batten disease, managing symptoms and optimizing quality of life becomes critical. Nutrition plays a critical role in this management, providing potential benefits in supporting overall health and slowing the progression of the disease. As such, creating a purposeful diet customized for people with Batten disease is vital for their well-being.

Evaluating Every Person's Nutritional Needs:

A comprehensive assessment by healthcare professionals, such as dietitians or nutritionists, is necessary to identify any nutritional deficiencies or challenges and tailor the diet plan accordingly. Before creating a diet plan for an individual with Batten disease, it is important to consider various factors, including age, weight, height, level of physical activity, specific symptoms of the disease, and any comorbidities. Individuals with Batten disease frequently experience difficulties with eating, such as dysphagia (difficulty swallowing) or chewing problems, which can significantly impact their ability to obtain adequate nutrition.

Making A Meal Plan That Is Balanced:

For people with Batten disease, a well-balanced meal plan is crucial to ensuring they get enough nutrients while controlling their symptoms. This meal plan should consist of a range of nutrient-dense foods from all food groups, such as fruits, vegetables, whole grains, lean proteins, and healthy fats. Nevertheless, because eating and swallowing can be difficult for people with Batten disease, adjustments to the meal plan may be needed to make it more individualized. For instance, softened or pureed foods can be added to the diet to make eating easier. Additionally, adding foods high in antioxidants, vitamins, and minerals can help reduce the oxidative stress and inflammation associated with

Advice On Portion Control And Meal Preparation:

Meal preparation and portion control are essential aspects of managing a bowel disease diet effectively. It's essential to plan meals, taking into account any dietary restrictions or preferences, as well as individual needs and abilities. Meal preparation may involve batch cooking and freezing portions for later use, making it easier to ensure a consistent intake of nutritious meals despite any physical limitations or fatigue. Additionally, portion control is crucial to prevent overeating and maintain a healthy weight, especially considering that individuals with Batten disease may have reduced mobility and energy expenditure. Using smaller plates, measuring portions, and being mindful of portion sizes can help promote satiety and prevent excessive calorie intake.

Moreover, involving family members or caregivers in meal preparation and planning can provide much-needed support and assistance, fostering a collaborative approach to managing the dietary needs of individuals with Battens Disease.

designing a diet plan for someone with Batten disease involves taking into account their unique nutritional requirements, coming up with a balanced meal plan, and putting strategies for meal preparation and portion control into practice. By taking these factors into account in a comprehensive way, people with the disease can maximize their nutritional intake, effectively manage their symptoms, and enhance their general health and well-being. However, to guarantee that each person with the disease receives individualized, evidence-based dietary recommendations that are tailored to their specific needs, healthcare professionals—including dietitians—must be involved in the process.

CHAPTER 4
FOODS HIGH IN NUTRIENTS FOR BATTENS DISEASE

Batten disease is a rare neurodegenerative disease that primarily affects children.

Of the foods that are high in nutrients, fruits, and vegetables are the main sources of important vitamins and antioxidants. Eating a range of fruits and vegetables provides a spectrum of nutrients that are needed for general health and well-being.

Fruits and vegetables are high in vitamins like C, A, and various B vitamins, which are essential for immune system support and cellular function. They also contain a variety of antioxidants, such as flavonoids, carotenoids, and polyphenols, which help fight oxidative stress and inflammation, both of which are linked to the development of Batten disease. Therefore, emphasis

Lean proteins—fish, poultry, tofu, and legumes—provide essential amino acids required for immune system function, tissue repair, and muscle maintenance.

However, choosing lean protein sources is important to minimize the intake of saturated fats and cholesterol, which may exacerbate certain symptoms of the disease, such as cardiovascular complications. By prioritizing lean protein sources, individuals with Batten disease can ensure adequate protein intake while supporting their overall health and minimizing potential adverse effects. Not to be overlooked, lean proteins are essential for meeting protein needs while maintaining overall health in individuals with the disease.

Furthermore, healthy fats are of paramount importance in managing Batten's Disease. Despite the misconception that all fats are detrimental to health, certain fats are beneficial and necessary for various physiological functions. Healthy fats, such as monounsaturated and polyunsaturated fats found in foods like avocados, nuts, seeds, and fatty fish, provide essential fatty acids, such as omega-3 and omega-6, which are critical for brain health, inflammation regulation, and cellular membrane integrity. Incorporating these healthy fats into the diet can help support cognitive function and mitigate inflammation, both of which are significant concerns in Batten disease management. However, it is crucial to moderate the intake of unhealthy fats, such as trans fats and excessive saturated fats, as they can contribute to inflammation and cardiovascular complications, which may worsen the prognosis of individuals with Batten disease. Therefore, focusing on healthy fat sources while minimizing unhealthy fats is essential for optimizing nutritional strategies in Batten disease management.

to support overall health and well-being, people with Batten disease should adopt a diet rich in nutrient-dense foods. They should also emphasize fruits and vegetables, lean proteins, and healthy fats to ensure adequate nutrient intake while minimizing potential exacerbating factors. Finally, it is advisable to consult with a healthcare professional or registered dietitian to customize nutritional strategies to individual needs and maximize the results of disease management.

CHAPTER 5
AVOIDING TRIGGER FOODS AND SUPPLEMENTS

As a neurodegenerative disease that progresses, Battens Disease necessitates the management of symptoms through diet. One aspect of managing symptoms through diet is avoiding trigger foods and substances that may worsen the condition.

This means that one must understand the influence of specific dietary components on the progression of symptoms and overall health. Although trigger foods and substances vary from person to person, common culprits include those high in refined sugars, artificial additives, and certain allergens. Knowing the function of these triggers is critical in creating a deliberate diet plan that aims to reduce the severity of symptoms and improve the quality of life for those with Batten disease.

Recognizing Foods That Could Make Symptoms Worse

When it comes to managing Batten's Disease, it is critical to know what kinds of foods can exacerbate symptoms.

Certain foods can exacerbate inflammation, oxidative stress, and neuronal damage, which can accelerate the disease's progression. These foods include highly processed foods, trans fats, and refined carbohydrates, which can interfere with metabolic processes and cellular function.

In addition, people with Batten disease may have dietary sensitivity or intolerances to particular food groups, which can make dietary decisions particularly challenging.

The management of symptoms and general health in patients with Battens Disease depends on the identification and avoidance of potential allergens and sensitivities. Allergens can elicit adverse reactions in susceptible individuals by inducing inflammation and exacerbating neurological symptoms associated with the disease. Common allergens include gluten, dairy, and certain proteins found in nuts and shellfish.

Additionally, sensitivities to food additives, such as artificial colors and flavors, can worsen symptoms and impair overall health. Consequently, close attention to ingredient labels and allergen profiles is critical when creating a dietary plan that minimizes allergic reactions and maximizes nutritional support for Battens Disease patients.

Handling Food Preservatives And Additives

The management of food additives and preservatives is critical in the context of Batten disease management. Many processed foods contain artificial additives and preservatives, which can have negative effects on neurological function and general health. Some additives, like artificial sweeteners and monosodium glutamate (MSG), have been linked to neurotoxicity and the exacerbation of neurodegenerative conditions. Preservatives, like sulfites and nitrates, can cause adverse reactions in individuals with sensitivities or compromised metabolic pathways. Consequently, adopting a diet that prioritizes whole, minimally processed foods is crucial in minimizing exposure to these harmful additives and maintaining neurological function in Battens Disease patients.

a comprehensive approach to managing Batten disease through diet entails avoiding trigger foods and substances, comprehending possible aggravating factors, recognizing allergens and sensitivities, and controlling food additives and preservatives. Patients and caregivers can maximize nutritional support, reduce symptoms, and improve quality of life in the face of this difficult neurodegenerative disease by diligently and carefully putting these strategies into practice.

CHAPTER 6
FLUID INTAKE AND HYDRATION

Maintaining adequate hydration is critical for the proper functioning of cells, tissues, and organs as well as for the regulation of body temperature, elimination of waste products, and transportation of nutrients.

It is also important for managing Batten's Disease because dehydration can lead to complications like muscle weakness, seizures, and impaired cognitive function. Individuals with Batten disease may also find it difficult to swallow, have limited mobility, and be more susceptible to dehydration from medication side effects. So, knowing how important it is to stay hydrated is essential for maintaining overall health and well-being.

Maintaining adequate hydration levels is crucial in managing Batten disease and minimizing the burden of associated symptoms. Healthcare providers and caregivers play a vital role in educating patients and their families about the importance of proper hydration and maintaining overall health and well-being.

Dehydration can exacerbate symptoms like fatigue, muscle weakness, and cognitive impairment, further compromising the individual's quality of life.

Additionally, dehydration can increase the risk of complications like urinary tract infections and constipation, which can significantly impact the individual's comfort and health status.

Selecting appropriate beverages can significantly contribute to meeting hydration needs and supporting overall health in individuals with Batten disease. Water is the primary and most effective hydrating beverage, providing essential hydration without added sugars, calories, or artificial additives. Encouraging individuals with Batten disease to consume water regularly throughout the day can help maintain adequate hydration levels and prevent dehydration. Additionally, other hydrating beverages such as herbal teas, electrolyte drinks, and coconut water can be beneficial, especially for individuals who may have difficulty consuming plain water due to taste preferences or swallowing difficulties. However, it's essential to be mindful of added sugars, caffeine, and artificial ingredients in certain beverages, as these may have adverse effects or contribute to dehydration in some cases. Healthcare professionals can guide on selecting hydrating beverages that best suit the individual's preferences and nutritional needs.

Tracking Fluid Consumption For Optimal Health

Regular monitoring of fluid intake is essential for individuals with Batten disease to ensure they are adequately hydrated and prevent dehydration-related complications. Healthcare providers, caregivers, and individuals themselves should track daily fluid intake and urine output to assess hydration status effectively. Keeping a fluid intake diary or using smartphone apps can help individuals monitor their hydration habits and identify any patterns or trends that may indicate inadequate fluid intake. Additionally, incorporating strategies such as setting reminders to drink water regularly, using hydration aids such as straws or sippy cups for individuals with swallowing difficulties, and adjusting fluid intake based on environmental factors such as temperature and physical activity level can help optimize hydration status. Furthermore, healthcare professionals may recommend periodic assessments of hydration status through urine tests or blood tests to detect early signs of dehydration and intervene promptly. By implementing proactive monitoring strategies, individuals with Batten disease can maintain optimal hydration levels and support their overall health and well-being.

CHAPTER 7

PARTICULAR ASPECTS AND DIFFICULTIES

Individuals affected by Batten disease encounter a myriad of challenges and considerations, necessitating tailored approaches to address their unique needs. Among these challenges, swallowing difficulties stand as a prominent concern. Batten disease, a rare neurodegenerative disorder, progressively impairs various bodily functions, including swallowing.

As the disease advances, individuals may experience dysphagia, making it challenging to consume solid foods safely and efficiently. Swallowing difficulties not only impede nutritional intake but also poses significant risks such as aspiration pneumonia. Therefore, managing swallowing difficulties requires a comprehensive approach involving specialized assessments, adaptive strategies, and nutritional interventions. Speech-language pathologists play a crucial role in evaluating swallowing function and recommending appropriate techniques, such as modified food textures and swallowing maneuvers, to enhance safety and efficiency during meals. Additionally, dietary modifications, such as thickened liquids and pureed foods, may be necessary to accommodate swallowing impairments and minimize the risk of aspiration. Collaborative efforts between healthcare professionals, caregivers, and individuals with Batten disease are essential to implement effective strategies that optimize nutrition while ensuring safe swallowing.

Handling Symptoms of the Gastrointestinal

Gastrointestinal symptoms are prevalent among individuals with Batten disease and can significantly impact their nutritional status and overall well-being.

As a neurodegenerative disorder, Battens Disease affects various organ systems, including the gastrointestinal tract, leading to symptoms such as constipation, gastroesophageal reflux, and delayed gastric emptying. These symptoms can exacerbate nutritional challenges by impairing appetite, causing discomfort, and interfering with nutrient absorption. Effective management of gastrointestinal symptoms requires a multifaceted approach addressing both symptomatic relief and nutritional support. Pharmacological interventions, such as laxatives and proton pump inhibitors, may be prescribed to alleviate symptoms and improve gastrointestinal function.

Additionally, dietary modifications play a crucial role in managing gastrointestinal symptoms and optimizing nutrition.

High-fiber diets, adequate hydration, and smaller, more frequent meals can help alleviate constipation and promote regular bowel movements. Moreover, avoiding trigger foods and adopting dietary strategies to minimize acid reflux can mitigate discomfort and enhance dietary tolerance. Healthcare professionals specializing in gastroenterology and nutrition collaborate closely to develop personalized management plans tailored to the specific needs of individuals with Battens Disease, aiming to optimize gastrointestinal health and nutritional well-being.

Techniques For Preserving Nutrition As The Disease Advances

As Batten disease progresses, maintaining optimal nutritional status becomes increasingly challenging due to a combination of disease-related factors and functional limitations. Progressive neurodegeneration affects various aspects of nutrition, including appetite regulation, swallowing function, and metabolic processes, leading to compromised nutritional intake and increased risk of malnutrition. Therefore, implementing strategies to preserve nutritional status is paramount in mitigating the adverse effects of disease progression and optimizing overall health and well-being. A holistic approach encompassing dietary interventions, nutritional supplementation, and supportive therapies is essential to address the complex nutritional needs of individuals with advancing Batten disease. Diet modifications tailored to individual preferences, dietary tolerances, and swallowing abilities play a central role in ensuring adequate nutrient intake despite progressive functional decline. Calorie-dense foods and nutrient-rich supplements may be prescribed to compensate for increased energy expenditure and nutrient losses associated with disease progression. Furthermore, supportive therapies such as enteral nutrition or parenteral nutrition may be indicated for individuals unable to meet their nutritional requirements orally. Regular monitoring by a multidisciplinary healthcare team comprising physicians, dietitians, and allied health professionals is essential to assess nutritional status, adjust interventions as needed, and optimize outcomes throughout the disease course. By implementing proactive strategies aimed at maintaining nutritional status, individuals with Battens Disease can enhance their quality of life and potentially slow the progression of associated complications.

CHAPTER 8
SUPPLEMENTS AND MEDICATIONS

Understanding the complex interactions between these supplemental measures and prescribed medications is essential for effective disease management. Supplements and medications play a critical role in supporting patients' health and well-being in the management of Battens Disease, a neurodegenerative disorder with devastating consequences.

Supplements' Function In The Management Of Batten Disease

Supplements are important for managing Batten's disease because they help with nutritional deficiencies, support body functions, and may even slow down the progression of symptoms.

Because Batten disease is progressive, people who have it often struggle with nutrient absorption and metabolism because of compromised cellular functioning.

As a result, supplementation is necessary to make up for these deficiencies and keep their health at its best. Additionally, some supplements have antioxidant properties that can help reduce oxidative stress, which is one of the factors that contributes to the neuronal damage seen in Batten's disease. Patients may find that their energy levels, immune system performance, and general quality of life are improved with targeted supplementation.

Frequently Suggested Supplements

Several supplements are commonly recommended for individuals with Batten disease to address specific nutritional deficiencies and support physiological functions.

Among the frequently prescribed supplements are vitamins such as vitamin A, vitamin D, vitamin E, and vitamin B-complex. These vitamins play vital roles in various cellular processes, including energy production, immune function, and neurological health. Additionally, minerals like calcium, magnesium, and zinc are often supplemented to support bone health, muscle function, and enzymatic activities. Omega-3 fatty acids, particularly eicosapentaenoic acid (EPA) and docosahexaenoic acid (DHA) are also recommended for their anti-inflammatory properties and potential neuroprotective effects. Moreover, certain antioxidant compounds such as coenzyme Q10 and alpha-lipoic acid may be prescribed to mitigate oxidative stress and its detrimental effects on neuronal cells. However, it's essential to consult with healthcare professionals to determine the appropriate dosages and formulations of these supplements based on individual needs and medical considerations.

Supplemental And Medicinal Interactions

Understanding and managing interactions between supplements and medications are paramount in Batten disease management to prevent adverse effects and optimize treatment outcomes.

Certain supplements may interact with prescribed medications, affecting their absorption, metabolism, or efficacy.

For instance, vitamin K supplements can interfere with anticoagulant medications like warfarin, potentially leading to fluctuations in blood clotting levels and increased risk of bleeding complications.

Similarly, calcium supplements may reduce the absorption of certain antibiotics, compromising their therapeutic effectiveness. Moreover, herbal supplements containing compounds like St. John's Wort can induce cytochrome P450 enzymes, which metabolize various medications, thereby altering their plasma concentrations and therapeutic effects.

To mitigate these interactions, healthcare providers must conduct thorough medication reviews and consider potential supplement-drug interactions when prescribing treatment regimens for Batten disease. Patients should also be educated about the importance of disclosing all supplement use to their healthcare team to ensure safe and effective disease management.

Additionally, close monitoring of patients' clinical responses and laboratory parameters is essential to detect and address any adverse interactions promptly. Collaborative efforts between patients, caregivers, and healthcare professionals are essential in navigating the complex landscape of supplement-medication interactions and optimizing therapeutic outcomes in Batten disease management.

CHAPTER 9
PRACTICAL ADVICE FOR CAREGIVERS

Batten disease is an uncommon and progressive neurological disorder that requires caregivers to manage a patient's daily activities, ensure their comfort, and tend to their medical and nutritional needs. Practical tips for caregivers cover a wide range of strategies targeted at improving the quality of life for both the patient and the caregiver. These strategies typically center around establishing a supportive environment, encouraging effective communication, and putting coping mechanisms into practice to deal with the challenges that come with providing care.

Caretakers may need to make adjustments to the home environment, such as installing grab bars, ramps, or specialized equipment to assist with mobility and accessibility. Establishing a routine schedule for daily activities can help provide structure and stability, reducing stress and anxiety for both the individual with Batten disease and their caregiver. Ensuring the safety and well-being of individuals with Batten disease is a crucial part of providing care.

Another important aspect of caregiving is emotional support. Batten disease can have a significant impact on the emotional and psychological well-being of both the affected person and their caregivers. To cope with the challenges of the disease, caregivers must be empathic, patient, and understanding. They must actively listen to the affected person's worries and feelings, providing comfort and reassurance when needed. Caregivers must prioritize self-care and seek out support from friends, family, or support groups to avoid burnout and maintain their own mental and emotional well-being.

Strategies for Meal Planning and Preparation

As the disease progresses, meal planning and preparation strategies become more crucial for individuals with Batten disease to maintain optimal nutrition and overall health. Appropriate nutrition can help slow down the disease's progression, alleviate symptoms, and improve the individual's quality of life. However, given the specific dietary requirements and restrictions associated with Batten disease, meal planning, and preparation can present significant challenges for caregivers.

A good way to plan meals is to concentrate on foods that are high in nutrients and contain vital vitamins, minerals, and antioxidants. These foods include fruits, vegetables, whole grains, lean proteins, and healthy fats. Caregivers should also try to include a range of foods from different food groups in the individual's diet to make sure they get enough nutrients. Finally, it's important to take the individual's preferences and dietary restrictions into account when meal planning. For example, some people with Batten disease may have trouble chewing or swallowing, so food textures or consistency must be adjusted. Other individuals may have particular food aversions or sensitivities that must be taken into account.

The way that meals are prepared can also have a big impact on how much nutrition is consumed by people with Batten disease. To make food easier to swallow or digest, caregivers may need to try different cooking techniques like pureeing, blending, or softening it.

In certain situations, commercial thickeners or supplements may be suggested to improve the nutritional value of meals. Finally, caregivers must collaborate closely with healthcare providers and nutritionists to create personalized meal plans that suit the needs and preferences of the individual.

Taking Care Of Dietary Challenges And Preferences

Managing dietary preferences and challenges is a critical component of optimizing nutritional intake for individuals with Batten disease. Patients may encounter changes in taste, appetite, and swallowing function, which can make it difficult to follow a balanced diet. Furthermore, the disease may progress over time, requiring modifications to the patient's dietary preferences and restrictions. Caregivers are essential in assisting patients with these challenges and making sure they receive enough nutrition to support their overall health and well-being.

Incorporating favorite foods or well-known dishes into meals can help make dining more pleasurable and fulfilling for the individual. Caregivers can offer a variety of options and encourage the individual to try new foods or flavors to stimulate their appetite and interest in eating.

Additionally, involving the individual in meal planning and decision-making can help empower them to make choices about the foods they enjoy and feel comfortable consuming.

Caregivers should be aware of any food allergies or sensitivities that the person with Batten disease may have and take precautions to avoid potential allergens or irritants in their diet.

In cases where people with Batten disease have trouble swallowing or chewing, it may be necessary to modify the texture or consistency of foods to make them easier to consume. This may involve pureeing, blending, or softening foods to create smooth or semi-solid textures that are safer and more manageable to swallow.

Seeking Assistance From Dietitians And Medical Professionals

When it comes to managing Batten disease and putting effective dietary strategies into practice, caregivers must enlist the help of nutritionists and healthcare professionals. These professionals, such as occupational therapists, dietitians, neurologists, and speech therapists, are vital in determining the individual's nutritional status, spotting potential problems, and creating interventions that are specifically designed to meet their needs.

 In addition to offering practical advice on ingredient selection, portion control, and meal preparation techniques to maximize the nutritional content of meals, nutritionists can collaborate with other members of the healthcare team to coordinate care and ensure a holistic approach to managing Batten disease. Nutritionists can provide invaluable guidance and expertise in creating customized meal plans that meet the individual's nutritional requirements and preferences.

Caregiver support groups can offer a safe and understanding space for caregivers to express their concerns, share experiences, and learn from others facing similar challenges. By forging strong connections with other caregivers and seeking support from healthcare professionals and nutritionists, caregivers can augment their capacity to provide effective care and support for individuals with Batten disease. In addition to professional support, caregivers may also benefit from connecting with other caregivers and support groups for mutual encouragement, information sharing, and emotional support.

CHAPTER 10
DIETARY MONITORING AND ADJUSTMENT

For those who suffer from Batten disease, diet management is essential. This is because neurodegenerative disease puts a great deal of strain on the body's capacity to absorb and use nutrients, so dietary management is a critical component of treatment. The basis of dietary management is routine nutritional assessment, which enables medical professionals to determine the patient's nutritional status, spot excesses or deficiencies, and customize dietary interventions.

The Value Of Continual Nutritional Evaluation

To effectively manage Batten disease, patients must have regular nutritional assessments. This is because the condition is progressive and has an impact on several bodily functions, including metabolism and nutrient absorption. An evaluation of the patient's nutritional status should be conducted regularly, and this can be achieved by reviewing their dietary intake, biochemical markers, anthropometric measurements, and clinical indicators. By doing so, healthcare professionals can identify any deviations from optimal nutritional status, such as deficiencies in essential vitamins and minerals or imbalances in macronutrient intake. By identifying nutritional issues early on, there is less chance of complications and the patient's overall health is optimized.

Identifying Symptoms Of Nutritional Excesses Or Deficiencies

Identifying signs of nutritional excesses or deficiencies in people with Battens Disease is one of the main goals of routine nutritional assessment. The disease's complex effects on metabolism and organ function make patients more susceptible to a variety of nutritional imbalances, which can show up in a variety of ways. For example, fatigue, weakness, poor wound healing, cognitive decline, and weakened immunity are examples of nutritional deficiencies, while excessive intake of certain nutrients, like fat or sodium, can worsen neurological symptoms or lead to cardiovascular complications. By closely monitoring clinical signs and symptoms in conjunction with objective nutritional markers, healthcare providers can identify the underlying nutritional imbalances.

Making The Diet Plan's Required Changes

Once nutritional deficiencies or excesses are identified, making necessary adjustments to the diet plan becomes imperative in managing Batten disease. These adjustments may involve modifying the composition of the diet to ensure adequate intake of essential nutrients while minimizing the risk of nutrient excesses.

For instance, individuals with Batten disease may require higher doses of certain vitamins or minerals to compensate for impaired absorption or increased metabolic demands. Similarly, dietary restrictions may be warranted to mitigate the adverse effects of nutrient excesses on overall health.

Collaborative efforts between healthcare providers, dietitians, patients, and their caregivers are essential in developing personalized dietary plans that accommodate individual needs and preferences while addressing nutritional concerns effectively.

Moreover, ongoing monitoring and reassessment are essential to evaluate the efficacy of dietary interventions and make further adjustments as needed, ensuring optimal nutritional support throughout Battens Disease.

 diet monitoring and modification are critical components of managing Batten disease and enhancing the health and well-being of those impacted.

 A key component of this process is routine nutritional assessment, which allows medical professionals to quickly detect nutritional excesses or deficiencies.

By identifying signs of nutritional imbalances and modifying the diet plan accordingly, healthcare teams can maximize nutritional Intake, minimize complications, and enhance the overall quality of life for patients with Batten disease.

It is imperative to stress the significance of continuous monitoring, teamwork, and individualized care to achieve optimal nutritional support and maximize therapeutic outcomes in this demanding clinical context.

CHAPTER 11
HOLISTIC APPROACHES AND LIFESTYLE FACTORS

Dietary interventions alone may not be sufficient to manage the complexities of Batten disease, so lifestyle factors become essential components of a holistic care plan. Lifestyle factors are important in the management of Batten disease, a rare neurodegenerative disorder with significant implications for quality of life. Holistic approaches encompass a comprehensive understanding of the interplay between various facets of an individual's life and health, seeking to address not only the physical symptoms but also the emotional and psychological well-being of patients.

Exercise and physical activity are vital components of holistic management for people with Batten disease.

Although the disease's course may eventually make mobility difficult, customized exercise programs can help sustain cardiovascular health, muscle strength, and flexibility for as long as possible. Exercise also encourages the release of endorphins, which can help reduce symptoms of anxiety and depression that are frequently associated with chronic illnesses. Finally, regular exercise builds a sense of empowerment and control over one's body, which is especially beneficial for people who are coping with the challenges that come with Batten disease.

For people with Batten disease and those who care for them, stress management techniques are essential.

The unrelenting course of the disease and the uncertainties that accompany it can result in elevated levels of stress and anxiety. As such, implementing strategies for managing stress becomes critical to preserving general well-being.

Methods like progressive muscle relaxation, mindfulness meditation, and deep breathing exercises can reduce stress and foster a sense of calmness.

Seeking social support via support groups or counseling can offer emotional comfort and useful coping strategies for navigating the emotional rollercoaster that is Batten's disease.

Alternative medicine and complementary therapies provide further avenues for a comprehensive approach to managing Batten disease; however, they should not be used in place of standard medical care because they address aspects of health that traditional medicine alone is unable to fully address. Acupuncture, massage therapy, and aromatherapy are examples of practices that have shown promise in addressing symptoms like pain, stiffness in the muscles, and sleep disruptions that are frequently experienced by patients with neurodegenerative diseases.

Additionally, certain dietary supplements may provide neuroprotective benefits or assist in addressing specific nutritional deficiencies linked to Batten disease.

CONCLUSION

By embracing a holistic care plan that takes into account the interconnectedness of physical, emotional, and psychological health, individuals with Batten disease can strive for improved quality of life and better symptom management.

Taking a holistic approach to managing the disease involves addressing lifestyle factors beyond dietary interventions alone.

These factors include incorporating physical activity and exercise, implementing stress management techniques, and investigating complementary therapies and alternative medicine.

www.ingramcontent.com/pod-product-compliance
Lightning Source LLC
Chambersburg PA
CBHW050655250726
48662CB00002B/694